D1596024

Honey, I Sold the Red Cadillac

Learning to Cope With Lewy Body Dementia

Bob Wolf

Table of Contents

Prologue

This is a true story describing various episodes in Bob and Carol's meandering path as they learned to cope with the onset and development of Lewy body dementia (LBD). It is written in the first person, from Bob's perspective.

First, a brief description of LBD. It is a progressive, degenerative disease that has some similarities with both Parkinson's disease (PD) and Alzheimer's disease (AD).

According to WebMD, PD is a chronic, progressive, degenerative disease characterized by motor symptoms that include tremors, muscle stiffness, and slowed movement. About a third of patients also develop dementia during later stages. One study, reported in 2010, indicates that the period from the onset of physical symptoms to the time to death may range from 2 to 37 years.

Alzheimer's disease (AD) is also a degenerative disease. The average life expectancy after diagnosis is 8 to 10 years; it can be as short as 3 years or as long as 20 or more years. But it can go undiagnosed for several years.

People with LBD exhibit some of the motor problems of PD (tremors, freezing, micrographia, or the gradually decreasing size of letters as one writes a sentence, and so on) as well as hallucinations, which typically occur in the later stages of PD. They also exhibit some memory issues commonly associated with AD. For people with LBD, life expectancy is short: 2 to 7 years after diagnosis. However, LBD is seldom diagnosed until well into the disease process. Life expectancy from the first LBD symptom remembered by spouse or family would likely be similar to AD's 15 to 20 years—perhaps longer with good care.

The First Symptoms

Our grandson was born in October 2002. In early in 2003, we were babysitting our grandson. He was crying, and we quickly discovered that the reason for his complaint was a thoroughly soiled diaper. That was not our only discovery on that fateful day. After making the child comfortable, Carol reported that she was unable to smell the mess. Although this may seem like an asset for a babysitter, the inability to detect odors is a detriment in day-to-day life. We decided to try to learn why her sense of smell had suddenly been turned off.

Our general practitioner (GP) ran several tests, the results of which were all negative. He then referred us to an ear-nose-throat (ENT) specialist, who ruled out a blow to the head, other traumatic events, or an olfactory problem. After several other tests, the ENT, too, could not identify the cause of the problem.

Neither physician mentioned the possibility that Carol's symptom might be an early indication of PD. Much, much later (in the fall of 2010, after Carol had been originally diagnosed with PD), we learned that loss of smell is a symptom commonly experienced by many PD patients. It is not clear whether our two doctors were not aware of the relationship between PD and loss of the sense of smell or just did not make the connection.

Fast forward to March 2010. Carol underwent surgery to repair a problem with the rotator cuff in her shoulder. After such surgery, physical therapy (PT) typically lasts for approximately 6 months. Once Carol had completed her last PT session in the fall of 2010, she visited the surgeon for a final checkup. Everything was fine; full mobility was restored to her arm and shoulder. As the visit was about to end Carol casually mentioned that earlier in the week, as she was reaching to turn off a bedside lamp, she felt a tremor in her left arm. The surgeon indicated that there were various possible causes for this and then went on to ask her a series of questions, including one about micrographia. Carol's handwriting had been deteriorating for some time.

The surgeon then suggested that Carol make an appointment with a neurologist.

(Note: Much later, at a Parkinson's Support Group meeting, we learned that people diagnosed with PD should, if at all possible, avoid surgeries that involve anesthesia, as this tends to worsen the physical symptoms of PD. The timing of Carol's first tremor leads me to conclude that Carol probably had tendencies toward PD but that they were accelerated by the anesthesia administered for her rotator cuff surgery.)

The neurologist ran several typical tests and concluded that Carol was indeed suffering from PD.

The Learning Process Begins

After Carol's diagnosis, she began participating in PT sessions specifically tailored for people with PD. I don't know if they did any good; but they didn't do any harm, so she continued them. She attended those classes for several months.

We also began attending the meetings of a local Parkinson's support group, where we met a physical therapist who specialized in treating patients with PD. After the meeting, we took him aside to ask him what could be done to minimize the problems Carol was beginning to have with walking. He then took us into an empty room and watched Carol walk.

He asked Carol to stand in the middle of the room and estimate how many steps she would have to take to reach a side wall. She said 14, and started walking and counting her steps. Interestingly, her steps were not the typical half steps that she had been taking and that are common to many people with PD. They were normal-sized steps.

When she had counted 11 steps and was clearly not going to make it in 14, she took three very, very long steps, just to be able to reach the wall in the predicted number. I would have wagered a lot of money that Carol would not be able to do what I had just seen her do. I would have lost that bet.

The physical therapist explained that walking is normally a semiautomatic activity. We don't really think about it as we do it. The activity of walking is triggered by a part of the brain that is involved in PD and affected by the loss of dopamine, which impacts the body's ability to send messages from the brain to a particular muscle. This explains the shuffling walk typically seen in patients with PD. However, when we superimpose the physical activity of walking on the mental activity of counting steps, the walking is triggered by a different part of the brain, unaffected by loss of dopamine, so walking is once again closer to normal.

I have guided Carol through that process of counting her steps many, many times since then. The process *always* works; she always walks more normally.

We Move to a New Home

(Medication note: In July 2011, Carol began taking amantadine to improve her mobility. Her soft voice and penmanship were not altered by the medication, and she began exhibiting a forward-leaning posture.)

During the summer of 2011 we were still living in Lafayette, California, although we were preparing to move. Our house was located at the end of a cul-de-sac on a street of only six houses. Next door lived a family with two high-school-aged boys and a dog.

In the process of preparing our house for sale, we had replaced the fence between our house and the neighbors' house with a new one. We also installed a gravel path leading from the gate into our backyard. We had the backyard landscaped and asked a landscaper to put in a new lawn.

Late one night, as we were lying in bed preparing to go to sleep, Carol said she heard the neighbor boys running down our gravel path. From the window I couldn't see anyone, so I took a flashlight and went out the back door for a better look. I didn't see any signs of anyone, and the gate was closed. This event (or nonevent) was repeated for several consecutive nights and then stopped.

A few nights later, Carol reported that she could see a large vague figure (perhaps 10 feet tall) in the bedroom, looking something like Paul Bunyan. This experience recurred every few nights, on each of which Carol saw a different large figure. The figures did not seem threatening and Carol wasn't frightened by them, but she did find it unusual and somewhat disturbing.

During that period we were quite preoccupied with selling our house. After it was sold, we were similarly engrossed with buying a new home, to the extent that Carol's visions faded to the background.

As part of the analysis and treatment of PD (and Carol's expressed concern about symptoms of AD), the neurologist suggested that Carol undergo a neuropsychological evaluation. The test was administered in August 2011, and she performed very well in most of it.

In July 2011 we made an offer on a home a few miles away in the senior community of Rossmoor , and on August 30, 2011, we moved into our new home.

Things Start to Get Interesting

Our new home has a dining room that looks out onto the entry of the house, and beyond that a tree and some shrubbery can be seen.

Shortly after we moved in, Carol began telling me about various things that she saw outside our dining room window. One day she described in great detail a circus that had been set up in our yard. Of course I couldn't see it. Another day she told me about several fire trucks parked by our garage. I looked out the window and saw nothing. A few days later she described a wedding that was taking place, again outside our dining room, complete with a bride in a white wedding dress. Days later, she reported that a group of children were playing in our yard. The reader must understand that Rossmoor is a senior community with virtually no residents under the age of 50.

Carol was also concerned that the nursery school near the far end of our building was very noisy, and that the little children were running wild.

Then there were the animals. Once she saw a little dog standing on its hind legs on our patio. On another occasion she noticed a cat hiding behind our couch. Another day there was a small rodent scurrying around our living room. Carol was also concerned that the artificial plant in our living room was dying and losing its leaves; perhaps we needed to water it. Another time the same artificial plant was supposedly growing new leaves.

At about the same time Carol said that there was a restaurant in the next building. Although I tried to explain that Rossmoor had only one restaurant, located in the Creekside Clubhouse, she insisted that there was one next door and she wanted to try it out. Whenever she mentioned that, I would try to divert her by changing the subject.

The master bedroom in our new home has a sliding door covered by roman shades. Unfortunately there was a small gap between the end of the roman shade and the edge of the door. Carol was concerned that people standing on our porch could look in through that gap and spy on us. To alleviate her concern, I installed an adhesive window film to cover the entirety of both the sliding glass door and the bedroom window. That didn't ease her mind. She thought that people could still see through the window film.

I then took a bedsheet, attached it to the wall above the roman shades, and used masking tape along both sides of the sliding glass door to seal the opening. In spite of that, Carol reported that at night she would hear "workmen" on the patio outside our bedroom; she was concerned that they might still be able to see in. I couldn't convince her that this wasn't possible.

At a meeting with her neurologist that December, Carol complained that her hallucinations were occurring every night, disturbing her sleep, and also that her walking was becoming more awkward as the day progressed. Also at about that time, in mid-December, she had cataract surgery. Fortunately cataract surgery does not require general anesthesia and there were no ramifications as far as I could tell.

In December or January Carol began seeing bugs. First she said that there were bugs on her plate, so I tried wiping the plate clean. Then she saw bugs on the plates stacked in the cabinet. I ran all the dishes through the dishwasher, but bugs did not go away.

On January 2, 2012, Carol sent an email to her neurologist. Part of it read:

> Prior to being diagnosed with Parkinson's I had some occasional hallucinations. I started having nightly hallucinations sometime after I began taking amantadine. Recently I began having hallucinations both day and night. Now my hallucinations never stop. Mostly, they take the form of thousands of (ant-like) bugs crawling on walls, furniture, and even people. These ant-like creatures are in EVERY room of the house, the washing machine, the clothes closet, EVERYWHERE. I have even eaten a few of them unintentionally. NO ONE ELSE CAN SEE THEM.

She and I were both very concerned about these visions.

The Diagnosis Changes

Carol began taking quetiapine (Seroquel) on February 1, 2012, to control the hallucinations. She stopped taking it 2 weeks later because it decreased her mobility but did not affect the hallucinations, which had only become more frequent in the interval. The neurologist then prescribed olanzapine (Zyprexa). After 2 weeks on one pill a day, he increased the dose to two a day.

Immediately after beginning on the increased dosage, Carol began to fall. Although she had not fallen even once in the previous 6 months, she now fell every couple of hours. We could not reach her neurologist right away, so we met with her GP. He took her off olanzapine after she had been on it for 3 days. By that time she was black and blue from her waist to her ankles.

We were faced with a dilemma. If Carol took a medication to improve her mobility and to ease the Parkinson's symptoms, the hallucinations got worse. If she took medications to alleviate the hallucinations, the physical symptoms got worse. There was no way to alleviate both kinds of symptoms at the same time.

On March 2 Carol had an appointment for a follow-up neuropsychological examination. I went with her. In the interim between the first and second appointments with the neuropsychologist, I had kept a log to record Carol's hallucinations, and I took the log with me. There were entries every day, describing the hallucinations for that day. The following is a sample, which represents just two entries from that log:

2/15/2012 7:30 AM: men were here but just for a short time. 10 AM: thousands of bugs in every room in the house. Late afternoon saw children playing & sitting on wall outside neighbor's yard (there is no wall there). Around dusk: woman outside living room, inserted her hand inside and deposited a box of bugs in the living rm. 8 PM: person outside (Carol asked him to leave). Cat in living rm. 9 PM: someone outside closed bedroom sliding door cutting roman shades. Big spiders in purse & on floor. Around 9:30 (in bedroom): woman stuck hand through wall and deposited box of bugs in bedroom. Carol asked them to leave, then sprayed with insect spray. They stopped for a bit, then started depositing bugs again. While we were watching TV (from 9:30 to 11 PM) she heard voices outside bedroom.

2/16/2012 Around 7 AM: Carol saw thousands of bugs on wall and curtain, and on floor while walking to bathroom. Carol did not want me to leave the room until she had come back from the bathroom. After lunch: girl kneeling outside kitchen door. All types of bugs in house throughout the day. At dinner she saw bugs in her salad. When we returned from shopping (about 8 PM) Carol saw a masked girl working on wires in the garage. In the house a man ran past her on the way out. Then she saw an animal on its back on the fireplace mantle (sleeping) and said that dried hydrangeas in a wreath above the fireplace had been eaten. 3 or 4 people talking outside our bedroom door.

The hallucinations occurred every day for several weeks. These were the log entries for only two of the days.

Based on her tests and the descriptions of the hallucinations, the neuropsychologist's conclusion was that Carol had Lewy body dementia (LBD), *not* Parkinson's disease (PD). The difference between traditional PD and LBD (which is one of several variants of PD) is that people with PD will not have hallucinations for 15 or more years after the onset of physical symptoms. If hallucinations start at the same time as physical symptoms or before that, the disease is LBD.

Later, in March 2012, Carol was referred to a neurologist at the University of California, San Francisco, for a second opinion. This neurologist confirmed the diagnosis of probable LBD and recommended that she use a rolling walker to increase her stability. At this point the diagnosis was only "probable" LBD because there is no definitive test for the disease. For 18 months Carol had been treated as a PD patient, with no one realizing that the real problem was LBD and the hallucinations that accompany it.

Syncope

On February 6, 2012, Carol had an eye exam. She was in the middle of one of those very typical vision measurements commonly used to determine the prescription for glasses: "Which is clearer A or B?" when she suddenly lost consciousness for a few seconds. Because she came to almost immediately and exhibited no aftereffects, neither of us thought much about it. We didn't associate it with anything specific.

Less than a month later, Carol awoke one morning, walked across the room, sat down in a chair, and almost immediately passed out again, this time with loss of bladder control. Again she was unconscious for just a few seconds. This time we immediately went to see our local GP. He diagnosed it as a possible seizure but recommended no action.

Then again, on April 10, Carol lost consciousness and bladder control. We discussed it with the neurologist, who stated that most likely it was an episode of syncope. One definition of syncope is "A short loss of consciousness and muscle strength, characterized by a fast onset, short duration, and spontaneous recovery (otherwise known as fainting). It is due to a decrease in blood flow to the entire brain, usually from low blood pressure." The doctor's conclusion was that since Carol's blood pressure is normally low and blood pressure typically decreases when one rises from a horizontal position, such fainting episodes are not surprising. He recommended that she increase the salt intake in her diet, as that has a direct effect on blood pressure. This became a delicate balancing act, because I have a tendency toward high blood pressure and have generally tried to reduce the salt in the foods we consume. We compromised by having Carol drink tomato juice or V-8 juice, both of which are high in salt, and adding salt to her meals but not to mine.

Fortunately Carol has not experienced an episode of syncope since then. It is my totally unscientific opinion that Carol's body was just reacting to the multiple changes in medication that were taking place at that time. These were as follows:

February 1, started quetiapine (Seroquel)

February14, stopped quetiapine and started olanzapine (Zyprexa)

March 1, stopped olanzapine

April 16, started carpidopa/levodopa (Sinemet)

I believe that with all those changes, Carol's body just rebelled.

Variety in the Hallucinations

In February 2013 the teenage boys showed up in Carol's mental perception for the first time. Apparently they had put on some type of show, and (as she explained to me) when she did not tip them enough, they got angry. They would visit Carol most nights for many, many months and would behave in a threatening manner. One of their favorite activities was to pump bugs into the bedroom. They eventually began putting boxes over their heads, but Carol could still tell who they were.

Carol often heard trucks passing by our house. This is not surprising as we live on the main road that leads into and out of Rossmoor. She believed that they were slowing down and dropping off a group of workers or robbers who were going to invade our home. These men were often associated with the four teenage boys who were harassing her.

At the same time "workmen" began making alterations to the house, particularly the bedroom. They installed a system of pipes that ran along the walls close to the ceiling and dispensed gas into the master bedroom; Carol feared that we were going to be asphyxiated. Seemingly, Carol could hear the gas hissing when it was turned on. I tried going into the living room, returning to the bedroom, and telling her that I had turned off the gas. Sometimes that worked, sometimes it didn't. This continued for over a year.

The "workmen" installed cameras in the bathroom and in the dressing room. Cameras were also installed in the bedroom and began projecting images on the ceiling. They would take pictures of Carol sitting on the toilet or changing her clothes. Cameras were a disturbing presence for a long, long time. She was reluctant to go to the bathroom or to get dressed for fear that she would be photographed or filmed. She was convinced that the pictures would be posted on the Internet.

Next Carol began complaining about whole families spending the night in the house and sleeping in sleeping bags in the living room.

Among these "hallucinatory" people there was one woman who had taken a dislike to Carol. Carol reported that, for spite, this woman had removed a print that we had hanging in the master bath area and replaced it with a forgery. Another time this same woman had supposedly altered the colors on a LeRoy Nieman print that hangs in the dining room.

Earlier, while Carol was still able to quilt, she had made a quilt with penguins on it. This quilt was hanging over our bed. One day Carol insisted that it be taken down and hidden away because "they" were planning to steal it. I took it down and put it away but did not remove the mounting hooks. After a few days I asked her if it was okay to hang it back. When she agreed, I put it back up. Every couple of weeks this same routine was repeated: there would be a threat to steal or destroy the quilt, I would take it down, and days later I would rehang it.

Carol often described an elevator that was apparently located in our guest bathroom. It was necessary to take this elevator to reach the seventh floor (in our two-story building), where her boss or the vice-president of "the company" was holding a meeting that she had to attend. This would invariably result in an argument between us. I would ask her to show me the elevator; she would insist that it was there and that she needed to take it to get to this important meeting. I tried taking her outside and showing her that our building was only two stories high, so there could not be a seventh floor. As I discovered, being outside was a different world from being inside our unit. It could be a two-story building outside and still have seven or eight floors inside. Reality and rational thinking were not pertinent.

It evolved that the elevator was in the same place as the linen closet in the guest bath. I asked her to show me how it worked, but she could not figure it out. She insisted it was there and she had to take it to the seventh floor to attend that meeting. She would be quite adamant, and it would drive me up the wall. We never did get the elevator issue resolved.

One morning Carol awoke believing that we did not live in our house that but a family with two adults and one child lived there. It was a four-bedroom house (similar to our former home).

Another repeated hallucination was that the drapes were on fire. I went to the drapes and put my hand where the fire was supposed to be to show her that I was not being burned, but that changed nothing. The drapes were still on fire. I have since learned that other people with LBD have experienced this same hallucination.

Most disturbing was that Carol often had troubling dreams at night. She would awaken, remember the dream, and believe that it was reality. I could not convince her otherwise. Unfortunately the dreams were always scary and threatening.

I tried and tried to convince Carol that what she saw or heard was not real, all with absolutely no success. At a PD conference a year earlier I had been told that it was fruitless to try to dissuade someone from their hallucinations. As I learned, it is like beating your head against a wall. It feels much better when you stop. It was not until much, much later that I finally learned to accept Carol's reality as fact, or at least to allow her to believe that I accepted it.

In spite of what people say, variety is *not* the spice of life.

Caregivers

I first hired a caregiver in April 2012. At first the idea was that someone would be with Carol so that I could play bridge on Tuesdays.
Finding a caregiver was a challenge. I did not know anyone who
might serve in that role. We checked caregiver ads in the paper and
tried out two or three of them. None was appropriate.

Then a friend of Carol's mentioned a woman named Sharon who
worked in the same store where she worked. And Sharon agreed
to act as a caregiver on a part-time basis. She was about 10 years
younger than Carol and stayed with her while I played bridge. Carol
was still able to walk at that time, so they went shopping together,
chatted, and became friends. We kept this routine up through the
rest of 2012, all of 2013, and into March 2014. As time went on, Carol
became less able to move about unassisted and even needed help getting out of a chair or up out of bed. Unfortunately Sharon was a small
woman and, by early 2014, could no longer manage to help Carol,

though she weighed only 125 pounds (see the section on Sinemet, further on).

Sharon helped us to find the next caregiver, Molly, a Tongan woman, and much sturdier and stronger than Sharon. Unfortunately Molly did not drive, so she could not take Carol anywhere, but she was wonderful about seeing to all of Carol's needs. We also asked Molly to take on some housekeeping chores (dusting, vacuuming, laundry, and so on) at an increased wage, and she agreed. Up until then we had used a housekeeping service to handle these chores (but not the laundry). As a result, I was able to stop using the housekeeping service.

Unfortunately Carol viewed Molly as a housekeeper, not a caregiver. She complained to me about all the things that Molly had left undone. I am not sure if she had a clear view of how much assistance she needed in her day-to-day activities. By this time Carol not only had trouble getting out of bed but also needed help getting dressed and with most other daily chores.

Another problem was that if I was in the house, Carol would call me and not Molly for help. Finally, out of desperation and to get some quiet time for myself, I developed the habit of leaving the house as soon as Molly arrived and not returning until it was time for Molly to go home.

Starting in April 2014, Molly helped us 2 days a week, 7 hours each day. By June we had increased it to 3 days a week, 7 hours each day. This continued arrangement through the rest of 2014 and into 2015. In 2015 we again increased Molly's time to 4 days a week. This continued until Carol moved into an assisted living home mid-September 2015.

Falls

Sometime during 2012 Carol began falling occasionally (long after she had stopped taking olanzapine). It did not happen often, but always when I was not at home. Until that time I still felt comfortable leaving Carol alone. (Our notes from our visit to the neurologist indicate that in August 2012 she was falling about once a week.) When this happened, she would lose her balance, fall to the floor, and be unable to get up again. She would stay on the floor until I returned home, sometimes as much as a half hour later. I think these events distressed me more than they bothered Carol.

Whenever I went out to run an errand, I would worry all the time I was out about what I might find when I returned home. One time I noticed an ambulance driving up Rossmoor Parkway ahead of me, and as I drove I became more and more panicked. Fortunately it continued up the road past our entry, and everything was fine when I got home. But often I went through moments of extreme anxiety.

About that time we decided that Carol needed to start using a walker, a decision that was also based on the recommendation of a neurologist who had examined Carol. So we went to our local medical supply store and bought one. Carol was never very adept at using the walker, but it did inhibit her tendency to lose her balance and fall. She used her walker whenever she and Sharon went out shopping.

Note: in November 2013 Carol's neurologist prescribed a wheelchair, indicating that a walker was no longer a viable option.

The Sinemet Experience

On April 16, 2012, Carol's neurologist had prescribed Sinemet (a combination of levodopa to combat tremors and stiffness and carbidopa to calm the stomach). The plan was to start slowly (half a pill three times a day), and gradually, over a period of 10 days, to build up to a full dose of three pills a day. After she reached that dose, Carol began to become nauseated. We tried all kinds of remedies: ginger pills, rubbing her wrists, using sea-sick wrist bands, ginger ale—nothing worked.

After 2 weeks of daily bouts of vomiting, the neurologist prescribed an additional dose of carbidopa, which is supposed to calm the stomach in patients who are also taking levodopa. Stand-alone carbidopa pills are extremely expensive and almost impossible to find. I finally did succeed in finding them, but they had no effect on Carol's vomiting. I am now thoroughly experienced at cleaning up after a bout of vomiting (not something I wanted on my résumé).

This continued for a month, at which point Carol stopped taking Sinemet. During this time she lost over 30 pounds. After she stopped the Sinemet, the nausea gradually subsided and her appetite returned. NOTE: this is NOT recommended as a weight-loss diet!

This is not a knock on Sinemet. It's very good medication. But there is a right way and a wrong way to administer it. See the chapter titled "Rotating Neurologists" for a brief discussion of the right way to do it. Now, much later, Carol has been taking Sinement and benefiting from it for more than 2 years without any ill effects.

The Little League Baseball Team

By 2014 I was helping Carol with most activities of daily living: getting out of bed, dressing, going to toilet, and showering. Although for her going to the toilet was somewhat traumatic with those imagined cameras filming all the time, it was the showering that posed the biggest problem. By this time Carol could not stand unsupported. The master bath has a tub, so it was difficult for Carol to get into and out of the tub. We tried it only once. As a result, she had to use the guest bath, which has a shower but no tub. Fortunately there was no camera in the guest bath (I never asked Carol about that, fearing that if I mentioned it, one would appear). I purchased a plastic lawn chair (with arms) that I placed in the shower stall. I went into the shower with her and helped her lather up and rinse off, wash her hair, and so on.

The problems all began when Carol started hearing someone knocking on the bathroom door, asking to be let in while we were showering. This progressed to her feeling that someone was looking under the bathroom door. To stop that, I placed a rolled-up towel at the bottom of the door to block the gap between the door and the floor. It did not help. The knocking just became louder and more insistent . So she insisted that we hurry through the shower so that we could leave the bathroom as quickly as possible. It was difficult and frustrating to try to rush through a shower and still get her hair and body clean.

Then Carol said we could not take a shower because "the Little League Team" was planning on using the bathroom when they returned from their game. I am not sure who sponsored the Little League Team or why they chose our house to shower. At one point I told her it was okay for her to shower because the game was not going to be over for at least another half hour and we would be done by then. Again we hurried through the shower so we would be done by the time the Little League Team got there.

That began the ritual of scheduling Carol's showers so they would not conflict with the Little League Team's use of the bathroom. I told Carol that there was a schedule posted which outlined the use of the guest bathroom. I further told her that we had reserved the bathroom for whatever time I wanted her to shower. This helped us to get into the shower. I was still placing a towel at the bottom of the bathroom door to stop potential peeping toms from looking in on her. Of course, having scheduled the use of the guest bathroom did not prevent imaginary people from banging on the door and insisting that we hurry through the showering process.

This problem involving the Little League Team continued for months. Eventually it stopped. As with most hallucinations, I never knew what triggered it or what made it stop. During this period life was full of surprises; I just tried to accept them and cope to the best of my ability as they arose or went away.

Rotating Neurologists

In the fall of 2010, when the surgeon who had operated on Carol's rotator cuff suggested that she visit a neurologist, we asked our GP for a recommendation. He recommended a neurologist who had an office in the same building as his office. Carol saw this neurologist through the remainder of 2010 and all of 2011 and 2012. He guided her through the Seroquel/Zyprexa misadventure and the Sinemet fiasco. At the end of 2012 he moved his office some distance away and became very difficult to reach, so we asked for and got a recommendation for another neurologist.

The second neurologist was very personable and caring, even making house calls. He monitored the progression of Carol's illness through all of 2013. In November 2013, however, he informed his patients that he was no longer accepting insurance of any kind. We again needed to find another neurologist.

Fortunately, in late November, 2013, we attended a meeting of the local PD support group, where a neurologist made a presentation. We had already received the letter from our second neurologist and were on the lookout for a replacement, so I got her name and contact information and found out that she was accepting new patients. I called her office and got the next available appointment (April of the following year).

At that April meeting, our new neurologist informed us that Sinemet was the "gold standard" in Parkinson's medication and that she would get Carol on it with no problems. She was true to her word. Rather than 10 days, she prescribed a regimen that took 4 weeks to implement. But at the end of those 4 weeks Carol was taking three Sinemet pills daily with not a trace of nausea. The lesson we learned here was that Carol needed not just a neurologist but one who was a specialist in movement disorders. The only problem was that this neurologist was with the Parkinson Institute headquartered in Sunnyvale, a good hour's car ride each way if there was no traffic.

All was well for the rest of 2014. Then the neurologist announced that she was leaving the practice. But there were other movement disorder specialists at the Parkinson Institute who would see the patients in her practice, so in 2015 we began with neurologist number four.

Again we were fortunate. This physician was as good as or better than her predecessor. And she was reachable. We were happy campers. We discussed various medications with her, new research taking place in the field of movement disorder and dementia, and received good care.

Then this neurologist, too, decided to leave the Parkinson Institute and strike out on her own. She said we could continue to see her in the South Bay area, or she would recommend someone closer to home. We chose the second option. Our last appointment with her was in May 2016. We are now seeing neurologist number five, who is 10 minutes from Carol's assisted living home and also seems very competent.

The Broken Nose

On the morning of July 13, 2013, I was in the master bathroom going through my morning routine and Carol was in the adjacent bedroom walking toward the bed. Suddenly I heard a crash and turned to see Carol on the floor, bleeding from her nose. There was blood everywhere! In a state of panic I rushed over, grabbed something (I don't remember what), and applied some gentle pressure to try to stop the bleeding. Then I called 911. While waiting for the paramedics, I tried to make Carol comfortable, unlocked the front door, and started to mop up the blood.

After what seemed like forever but in reality was only a few minutes, a mass of people arrived. I believe there were two or three people from Securitas (the Rossmoor security people) and four paramedics. There may have been more people, but I have no recollection of it. The paramedics controlled the bleeding, loaded Carol into their ambulance, and left for the hospital.

I let everyone else out the door, locked up, and also left for the hospital. Somehow I managed to arrive at the John Muir Emergency Room before the ambulance. After Carol was off-loaded from the ambulance, she was checked in. The hospital had to find her records and make sure she was covered by insurance. Then they proceeded to examine her nose.

They determined that the nose was indeed broken but not out of place (the best of all worlds for a broken nose), so nothing needed to be done except apply ice periodically to control swelling. As long as it was not out of line, the broken bone in the nose would knit together of its own accord. The hospital released her at 1:30 that afternoon and I took her home.

Then I could begin breathing again (although my nose was fine).

Mealtimes

I had retired in 2002 and Carol continued to work for 3 more years. She worked as a systems analyst and project manager in a technology company dealing with emails. The company was located in Pleasanton, a community about a half hour away from our home in Lafayette. During that time we developed a routine wherein Carol would call me as she was getting ready to leave work, which would give me enough time to cook dinner.

Carol was not particularly fond of cooking and I enjoyed it, so it was a good arrangement. I tried to find interesting and tasty recipes that we would both like. At about that time our GP retired, and we started seeing a doctor who believes that a vegetarian diet is healthful. Some time later, when Carol was diagnosed with PD and I was doing some research on it, I discovered that a vegetarian diet is beneficial for people with PD. So we decided to become vegetarians. I found a great variety of recipes, mostly based on beans, that we particularly liked. Carol does not like tofu, so we avoided that.

Sometime around late 2014 or early 2015 Carol became a fussy eater. She refused to eat all the dishes she had previously liked. No matter what I prepared, she did not want to eat. Every meal became a battle. It was like trying to feed a 5-year-old child. I began dreading mealtimes. Somehow, in spite of the battles, we managed to find something that Carol would agree to eat at every meal.

Honey, I Sold the Red Cadillac

One morning Carol informed me that the teenage gang in the neighborhood was threatening to trash our red Cadillac. At this point it behooves me to point out that we don't own a red Cadillac, or any other color Cadillac—we have never owned a Cadillac of any color. Also, as we live in Rossmoor, a senior community, there are no teenagers in the neighborhood and certainly no gangs.

The next morning Carol told me that the teenagers had driven our red Cadillac into the creek. A couple of days later, I was alerted that the teenage gang had broken all the windows in our red Cadillac. Then, she complained that the teenagers had thrown trash into the red Cadillac. That was followed by the gang throwing paint all over our red Cadillac.

Finally, after several more days of a variety of catastrophic events befalling our beleaguered car, I told her one morning: "Honey, I sold the red Cadillac!" She had only one question to this revelation. She asked "How much did you get for it?"

My response was the only one that made any sense to me. I said "Blue Book."

Carol never mentioned the red Cadillac after that day.

That was an epiphany for me. I had come up with a response that calmed her fears. To do that I had to ignore the truth, move my brain into her altered reality, and deal with her concerns, threats, urgent situations, crises, and anything else that was troubling her in such a manner that it calmed her fears. I would use that tactic many times in the many months that were to come. I still use the technique, and it still works.

My Mother Is in the Hospital

Carol's mother died in 2008; she was cremated and her ashes were shipped to Warren Wilson College (in North Carolina). Carol and I went to Warren Wilson College and spread her ashes at the cemetery there. I have pictures of us at the cemetery and of the gravestone.

One day Carol said "My mother has been in a traffic accident and has been taken to the hospital. I need to go there and be with her." I tried to explain that her mother was dead. I showed her pictures of her mother's headstone and of us spreading he ashes. But Carol was adamant. She had to go to the hospital and be with her mother. This was a theme that I was to hear many times, with many variations.

At the time I could not think of a reason not to comply, so we got in the car and drove to the Muir Hospital emergency room. Of course, as I expected, they had no record of anyone with Carol's mother's name being admitted to the hospital, so we left and drove home.

A few days later, Carol reported that her mother had fallen down the stairs and had been taken to the hospital. This time I remembered the episodes with the red Cadillac. I went into our home office, came back a few seconds later, and told Carol that I had called the hospital. Her mother had been examined at the hospital. There were no broken bones, she had been bandaged up and sent home because she was fine. Carol was placated.

Another time Carol said that her mother had tripped, fallen down the stairs, and hurt herself. Again, a quick fictitious call to the hospital, and I was happy to report that there had been no damage. Again the hospital had released her and had sent her on her way.

The next time Carol informed me that her mother was in the hospital, I decided that the situation needed a slightly different approach. Carol's mother had been to the hospital and been fine too many times. This time I told her that this was a case of mistaken identity. Although the woman in the hospital had the same first name as Carol's mother, they had different last names. It was not her mother at the hospital at all.

Gradually, Carol's mother stopped going to the hospital.

Phone Calls From the Boss

At one time during Carol's working career she was employed by American Telephone and Telegraph (AT&T). Her responsibilities included providing technical support in the sale and installation of complex telephone systems. She had a good understanding of how they worked and the variety of systems available. As you will see, this became pertinent in one of her persistent hallucinations.

One morning Carol was in bed and told me she was talking to her boss (through the pillow). As she was not holding a telephone handset I asked how she was talking to him. She informed me that it was a special phone system that did not need the more traditional type of instrument to talk to someone. It also did not need wires. It was connected through the "company" operator and she could use it to reach anyone in the company.

This method of communication continued for over a year. She often received calls from her boss or the "company" vice-president calling her to a meeting. After a while, I learned that I needed to be quiet while she was on those phone calls, so as not to interfere with her ability to hear the other end of the conversation.

The calls evolved, and, after some time, Carol would hold these conversations while seated at the dining room table. She talked into and through the place mat on the table to whomever was on the other end of her imaginary phone call. Naturally I had to be quiet so she could hear the other end of the conversation.

One weekend, my son and our grandson were visiting from Los Angeles. At some point during their visit we were sitting at the dining room table, eating lunch, when Carol received a phone call on her fictitious phone system. My son and I were curious to see what my 5-year-old grandson would say—how would he react. He was not fazed by the event in the slightest. After all, he would habitually have fictitious telephone conversations with his friends or workers at his imaginary spying company. Those kinds of telephone conversations were a normal daily occurrence to him. He took it in stride. Normalcy is in the eyes of the beholder.

Getting Dressed

Carol needed help with most aspects of daily living. She needed assistance getting out of bed, going to the bathroom, brushing her teeth, getting dressed, showering, and so on. The only activity with which she did not need help was eating. In a subsequent chapter you will see why feeding herself became important.

We have a walk-in master closet, and shortly after we moved in we placed a chair and full-length mirror in the closet. During the ritual we developed, I would help Carol walk into the closet. She would then sit down on the chair and pick out the clothes she would wear for the day. As time went on, it took her longer and longer to decide what to wear. And on top of that she was always concerned that "they" were filming or taking pictures of her.

Carol informed me one morning that she needed to put on her fancy floor-length dress because she was getting married that morning. I tried arguing with her: "it's too fancy a dress," "save it for later," but nothing worked. She put it on. This scenario was repeated several times. Finally I stopped objecting. I decided that she could put on anything she liked. After all, what was she saving the clothes for?

Again I felt that I was raising a 5-year-old. She refused to eat her food, argued about what clothes to wear, knew how to push my buttons to get me angry. I found myself losing my temper more and more often. I didn't like the situation or my reactions to it.

One day she decided she needed to try on a number of different outfits. I don't remember why she needed to put on virtually every outfit she owned, but we started through the process. After she had put on about six different tops and pants, I finally lost my temper. I yelled at Carol and slammed the closet door, causing it to bang into Carol.

Instantly I regretted what I had done. I knew it was not her fault; she was not being difficult intentionally. I felt terrible. I apologized. I just could not undo what I had done. At that moment I knew something had to change. Carol's behavior was just wearing me out, and I didn't know what to do about it. After all, it was my responsibility to take care of her. We were married in 1984, and we had vowed: "to cherish and protect, in sickness and in health, for as long as we both shall live." I intend to keep those vows.

Moving Into Assisted Living

Early in 2015 Carol's daughter from an earlier marriage, Beth, started telling me that Carol should move into an assisted living residence. Living at home was not a good long-term solution. I insisted that I was quite capable of taking care of her. After all, I had help; a caregiver was coming 4 days a week for 7 hours a day, so I had 4 days off each week. How much more did I need?

Beth was not placated. She pointed out that I had 28 hours of help and there are 168 hours in a week, leaving 140 hours a week with no help. She also mentioned that something could happen to me—a debilitating fall, an illness that could hospitalize me, and on and on. Who would take care of her mom under those circumstances?

Unfortunately I had a very clear mental image of the home where Carol's mother had lived for several years at the end of her life. It was a very nice facility, with a lovely dining room where they served all the meals. I even had meals there with Carol and her mother on several occasions. But I also clearly remembered residents (mostly older women) lined up in their wheelchairs, sitting outside their bedroom doors. They would either sit there, asleep or staring into space, or occasionally crying for someone to help them. It was a very disturbing memory. I was *never* going to subject Carol to that kind of environment.

When I continued to balk at the idea, Beth scheduled a visit to one of the local assisted living facilities and asked me to go there with her. Reluctantly, I agreed. It seemed very nice: neat, clean, well run, and most importantly, no one was being ignored.

I decided that if I was going to consider this option (I was still not convinced), I should compare several available places. In the next week I visited five other facilities. I analyzed them, listed each place's good and bad points (I am hyperanalytical), and shared my analysis with Beth. Then I let the whole matter sit.

Pretty soon my daughter from an earlier marriage, Jessica, joined the chorus and started getting on my case about finding a place for Carol. By the end of August I had succumbed to their arguments. Jessica said that if I would reduce the list to two or three places, she would come with me to visit them. She lives in Brooklyn, New York, so it was not a casual offer. She arrived on Sunday. On Monday she, Beth, and I went to the top two places on my list. One of them, located in Lafayette, had no openings, but we were told of a sister facility, in Walnut Creek, that did have openings. Monday afternoon we visited that place and agreed that Carol should move there. Tuesday Jessica flew back to Brooklyn.

The next 2 weeks were spent buying furniture (most assisted living places provide an unfurnished room), arranging for delivery of the furniture and a hospital bed with a bed rail, and coordinating all that activity with Carol's future home.

The furniture and the hospital bed were delivered on September 15. The next couple of days were spent getting pictures hung, arranging to hang the penguin quilt that Carol had made, and buying a small TV set.

Finally the big day came. The move was scheduled for Saturday September 19. About a month earlier Carol had complained that she didn't have enough things to do. So on Friday I told Carol that I was going to take her to a resort with lots of activities in which she could participate. I clued in the director of the memory care unit, so when we arrived on Saturday, he greeted her with an effusive "Welcome to our resort!" and took her up to see her room and tour the premises.

The memory care unit in Walnut Creek consists of two floors connected by an elevator, with bedrooms on both floors as well as a common room and a dining room on each. The upstairs common room was like a living room and was used mostly for watching TV, typically movies. The downstairs common room was used for most other activities, including seated exercises and also watching TV.

For the next 2 months Carol lived at that facility, taking part in whatever activities they offered.

A Change of Venue

In November, 2 months after Carol moved into the Walnut Creek facility, I got a call from the director of the memory care unit telling me that there was a problem. I remember clearly that it was Friday the thirteenth. I went to the facility to talk with him in person. He told me that Carol was no longer able to feed herself, and that this was a problem because the facility was not staffed to offer feedings. I went to see Carol during a mealtime and saw for myself that this was really the case.

In short, it seemed that Carol would have to move out. The director also told me that another location of the same group, located in Lafayette, would have an opening the following Thursday. I had seen the Lafayette location during my initial visits to the nearby facilities—in fact, it was one of the three that Beth, Jessica, and I had all seen—and I had determined that it was more than acceptable. In fact, it was the place that had originally been full and had directed me to the one at Walnut Creek.

On Monday I went back to the Lafayette facility for a second look and to discuss space availability and support capabilities. They did indeed have a room that was to become available the following Thursday. By Monday Carol was again feeding herself, so I was left with a question: Do I leave her there and see if/when her feeding problem returns, or do I move her regardless of her condition? I decided to take the room while it was still available.

Now I had to find a furniture mover. After many phone calls I found one who could transport the furniture between facilities that same week. We settled on Friday. The next problem was one of space. The room in the new facility was smaller than the room she was currently in and had no TV connection. I decided to take the rocker, one night table, a lamp, and the TV to my home in Rossmoor and the rest of the furniture to the assisted living facility. The mover agreed to drop the furniture off at two separate destinations.

Next I had to arrange the timing of the move. I decided that the mover should arrive at Walnut Creek while Carol was at breakfast and move her furniture out at that time. After breakfast the staff would make sure that she stayed in the living room area, perhaps watching TV, without ever returning to her empty room. In the meantime I went with the movers to oversee the moving of the furniture to Lafayette and Rossmoor. I also arranged to have Carol's penguin quilt hung on the wall above the bed and the pictures of all the grandchildren hung on another wall.

Carol had had lunch at the facility in Walnut Creek, and after lunch I picked her up and took her to Lafayette. There she was shown her room (with all her things in it), and taken to the common room where music was playing. At 3 PM all the residents went up to the third floor for "Happy Hour." This is a Friday ritual where they have a musician play a guitar or the piano and sing familiar songs. They also serve a snack and punch.

I breathed a sigh of relief at the end of a highly stressful week.

As a final note to this episode, Carol has not experienced any trouble feeding herself in the year since her relocation. In fact, her physical and mental condition has deteriorated only slightly in all that time. If I were religiously inclined, I would say that God intervened to move her to a better place.

Who Am I

In talking with friends about Carol, I am often asked "Does she know who you are?" My usual response is "It depends." Most often I am Bob, her husband; but occasionally I am her father. I bear absolutely no resemblance to her father, who died in his sixties, when Carol was in her late twenties.

After giving it some thought, I finally realized that Carol's image of herself was that of a woman somewhere between 20 and 40 years of age. She is either a student, a young mother, or a working woman. I am an older man with white hair who makes all the decisions for her. Clearly I am her father.

Hallucinations

A curious thing happened after Carol moved into the assisted living facility in Lafayette. There was a change in the types of hallucinations that she was experiencing. Gone were those threatening, frightening hallucinations that she had been having at home. They were replaced by what I consider more benign hallucinations. In most cases she saw herself as a student in school, a young mother, or a woman in business.

When she is in the middle of one of those situations and becomes agitated, the caregivers at her new home will give her pencil and paper and get her started on a project in which she can visualize herself as being at work. She will sit, working on the imaginary project with paper and pencil for a long time.

I spend some time with Carol every day. One day I arrived at the facility and found her very agitated. She told me that she was responsible for arranging a trip for everyone in the group to fly on United

Airlines to Hawaii. Unfortunately United Airlines was giving her a hard time about paying for the flight or getting a refund for the flight—it wasn't clear which. I was amazed at the level of detail and specificity involved in the hallucination.

Once again I used the lesson of the Red Cadillac. I told Carol to leave the negotiations with United Airlines to me; I would deal with it. I stepped out of the room and waited about 5 seconds. Then I returned and told her that it was all resolved: United Airlines had agreed to refund all the money and the matter was settled. That calmed her down and we moved on to focus on whatever was scheduled as that day's activity.

The hallucinations continue, but they are nonthreatening. I don't know what caused the change; I only know that she is in a positive, upbeat environment where they have music playing all the time, and possibly that affects her mood.

The Birthday Party

One day Doris, Carol's new roommate, was celebrating her birthday. Or to put it more accurately, Doris's daughter had brought a sheet cake to the facility to celebrate her mother's birthday. I later learned that this is a standard ritual whenever a resident had local family to supply the cake. When I arrived to visit Carol, many of the residents were seated around a table and the cake was being served. As was my custom, whenever I arrived, I checked for Carol, and this time she was not in the common room.

I went into her bedroom, and found her lying in bed. I asked her if she wanted to join the group, but she said she was tired. So I left the room and approached Doris's daughter. She said she would be happy to have Carol join the group, so I returned to the bedroom and conveyed this invitation to Carol. She still said she did not want to participate because she didn't know anyone there.

Knowing how much Carol likes cake, I told her that Doris's daughter had specifically invited her and was in the process of cutting a piece of the birthday cake especially for her. Finally she agreed to take part in the celebration.

I helped her into the wheelchair (this was not a good time to have her struggle with the walker), and wheeled her out to the common room and to an empty space at the table. No sooner had she arrived at the table that she started to talk to one after another of the people at the table in a loud (for her) clear voice. It was as if she needed to get to know these people and was starting to "chat them up."

At that point I decided that Carol was involved and participating in the activity and it was an appropriate time for me to leave. I notched that up as a "good" day. I treasure the "good" days.

The Presidential Election

Sometime in mid-October our absentee ballots arrived, listing all the candidates and state propositions. Since we live in California, propositions are like mushrooms—give them an abundantly dark, moist environment and they will proliferate. This year there were 17 of them. The absentee ballots were followed shortly thereafter by the Voter Guide. This year it was a 228-page tome to be studied or ignored as voters chose.

After digesting all 17 propositions, I decided that it would be a good activity for Carol and me to discuss the ballot and actually fill it out. It would also give me an opportunity to assess Carol's state of mind. I gave Carol the names of the candidates for president and asked her who she wanted to vote for. She looked at me and said, "Hillary, of course. It's about time." Clearly women's rights are still as important to her as they always were.

We went through the remaining elective offices, with me providing a bit of guidance in the cases where Carol was not familiar with the candidates. After stepping through all the elective offices we turned to the propositions. Proposition 51 was about issuing bonds for school construction. Carol's reaction was "I am in favor of more money for schools—they can use it."

Carol may not know how old she is, what day of the week or month of the year it is, or whether I am her husband or her father, but some things are firmly fixed in her mind.

On Election Day the residents were sitting in the common room, as is their custom. The activities director started by asking one of the residents if she was going to vote. After asking two or three others, she turned to Carol and asked her the same question. Carol's reply was "No, Bob and I already voted."

Once again Carol had knocked me for a loop. I was firmly convinced that her long-term memory was fine but that she has essentially no short-term memory. Her answer proved that I was way off base. Filling out the absentee ballot was an important event that had registered with her.

Iceland

It was a Thursday. Every Thursday Carol and I go to Tremble Clefs to sing with other people who have PD, which causes their voices to get soft and low. Tremble Clefs was organized to provide Parkinsonians with an opportunity to exercise their voices by singing.

So this Thursday we went to Tremble Clefs. We were in the middle of rehearsing our winter holiday program, so many of the songs were Christmas carols that we already knew. As happens so often, during the first hour of rehearsals, Carol was attentive but not participating. She was just following along with the words of the various carols and complaining about a sore throat.

At the 2:30-PM snack break I gave Carol her Sinemet medication, which she usually takes at this hour. I don't know if the medication made a difference, but during the second hour of rehearsals she joined in and sang along for most of the songs.

When we returned to her home, the activities director was just starting to show the residents some travel slides from Iceland. She went through several photos of the countryside, the Aurora Borealis, wild horses, and molten magma. With each picture she would try to elicit some comment or reaction from one or another of the residents.

After six or seven pictures, she showed a picture of a beautiful church in the background, with a woman on ice skates on a frozen pond in the foreground. As the picture appeared on the screen, the activities director asked Carol "What is this woman doing?" Without missing a beat, Carol said: "Preparing to fall down!"

Final Thoughts for Others Traveling This Path

LBD is a debilitating disease—not just for the person afflicted with it but also for his or her loved ones and caregivers, particularly if the loved one is the primary caregiver. I have documented my experiences along this path in the hope that some of you will learn from my painfully acquired knowledge and perhaps that will make your travels down this treacherous and painful road a little easier.

First, a caveat: everyone suffering from LBD will experience it in a different way. But there are also similarities. I hope that you will read about one of the situations I have described and say "Oh! My loved one has experienced that episode." Or you will have read this and then run into a troublesome situation and ask "How did Bob deal with this?" I do not pretend to be the final authority on how these various circumstances should be handled, but I am presenting one option that you might want to consider.

Things I have learned:

1. Reality for your loved one is whatever he or she believes. It is not what you understand to be reality. Do not try to convince him or her otherwise. You will be wasting your breath. You will become frustrated. I cannot stress this enough.

2. Lying is not a sin, it is medication. It is problem solving. You are alleviating a symptom of the disease. You are helping to ease an afflicted mind. Problem solving (lying) gets easier with practice. It is a not-so-simple two-step process:

    a. What is the manifestation of the underlying problem? You may never learn what the real problem is, but how is it expressed?

    b. What can you say or do to ease the concern? Remember the *Red Cadillac*. I don't know what Carol was worried about, but I made the Cadillac go away and the problem was gone with it.

3. Take care of yourself first! Remember what you are told on an airplane: "Put on your oxygen mask before putting one on your child." You are your loved one's oxygen mask. If you are sick or otherwise unavailable, who will take care of your loved one? Care for yourself first, so that you'll be able to care for your loved one.

4. Pick a neurologist carefully. LBD is a very complex disease and quite different from PD. You need someone who is a movement disorder specialist and also understands

the ramifications of dementia and hallucinations. Don't be afraid to interview several prospective neurologists. Ask about their experience with this disease.

5. Life can get better. The disease and its symptoms will not get better, but day-to-day living can. Perhaps you have noticed that the chapters following Carol's move to a new venue are essentially upbeat. This was not accidental, although it was unexpected. Carol is living in a stimulating environment: music is playing at all times, a variety of activities (all designed to involve the residents) are presented every day, physical and mental exercises are offered. And, as a bonus, I have not lost my temper even once in the past year. When I spend time with Carol, we can enjoy being together.

6. Each person with LBD is different, and their symptoms manifest themselves differently, but there are similarities in the hallucinations. I have spoken with other caregivers who have mentioned drapes being on fire, invisible guests at their tables, and strange things happening to their paintings.

7. Talk about your experiences. Sharing helps. If you have LBD, join an LBD support group. If you can't find a local one, join a Parkinson's support group. There are a lot of symptoms that they share. If you are caring for someone with LBD, join a caregiver support group. Any dementia caregiver support group will do. There are many similarities in the experiences of caregivers for loved ones with all forms of dementia. Listen and talk. Both will help.

Final thoughts:

Acceptance does not occur overnight. It took me 6 months to accept, mentally, the idea of Carol living in an assisted living home; but once there, she was in a better place than I could provide. It took me a full year to accept that emotionally.

For anyone reading this who knows someone caring for a loved one with LBD, tell them you understand their pain. Do something nice for them.

If you are reading this and caring for a loved one with LBD, others have walked this same path. Others have gone through the same situations, others are going through these situations right now. You are not alone.

Good luck and Godspeed.

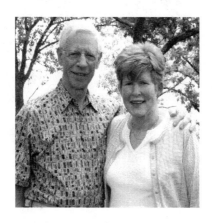

About the Author

Bob was born in Panama in 1937. He moved to Southern California with his family when he was 7 years old. After obtaining a Bachelor's degree in Engineering at UCLA and a Master's degree in Operations Research at NYU, he worked in the computer and telecommunications industry. While working at Pacific Telephone Co. he met Carol.

Carol had a Bachelor's degree from Wooster University and was in the first class of women admitted to the Master's program at Harvard University. After a two-year courtship they were married on Dec. 31, 1984. The marriage created a "Brady Bunch" family: three children from Bob's earlier marriage and two from Carol's first marriage.

Both Bob and Carol were retired and living in Lafayette, CA (a small town in Northern California) when Carol first detected a tremor in her left hand, foretelling the onset of Parkinson's disease. This was the start down that long twisting path that is described in this book.